The Definitive Thai and Oriental Dessert Drinks and Soups Cookbook

50 super easy and affordable Dessert, Drinks and Soups recipes for your Thai and Oriental food

Madeline Soto

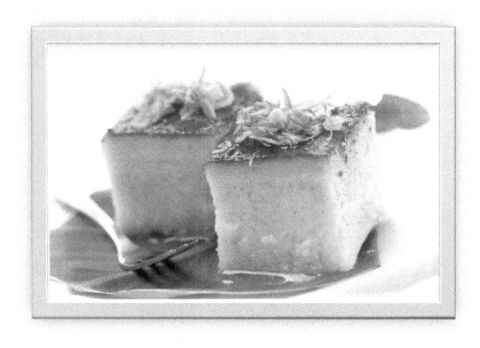

Table of contents

BANANA COCONUT SOUP

Ingredients:

1 cinnamon stick

1 tablespoon lemon juice

2 tablespoons minced gingerroot

4 cups banana slices, plus extra for decoration

4 cups canned coconut milk

Salt to taste

Directions:

1. In a big deep cooking pan, bring the coconut milk to its boiling point. Put in the banana, ginger, cinnamon stick, lemon juice, and a pinch of salt. Decrease the heat and simmer for ten to fifteen minutes or until the banana is very tender.

2. Take away the cinnamon stick and let cool slightly.

3. Using a handheld blender (or a blender or food processor), purée the soup until the desired smoothness is achieved.

4. Serve the soup in preheated bowls, decorated with banana slices and coconut.

Yield: Servings 6–8

BANANAS POACHED IN COCONUT MILK

Ingredients:

¼ teaspoon salt

1 cup sugar

2–3 small, slightly green bananas

4 cups coconut milk

Directions:

1. Peel the bananas and slice them in half along the length.

2. Pour the coconut milk into a pan big enough to hold the bananas laid flat in a single layer. Put in the sugar and salt and bring to its boiling point.

3. Reduce the heat, put in the bananas, and simmer until the bananas are just warmed through, approximately 3 to five minutes.

4. Serve the bananas warm on small plates decorated with fresh coconut and pineapple wedges.

Yield: Servings 2–3

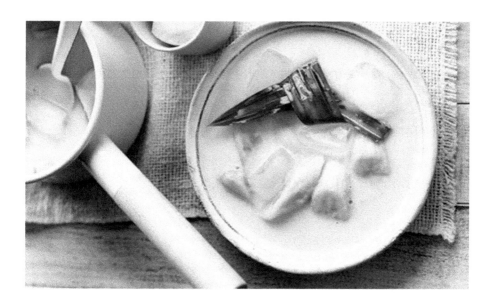

CITRUS FOOL

Ingredients:

½ cup heavy cream

½ cup orange, lime, or lemon juice

1 big egg, beaten

2 (3-inch-long, ½-inch wide) strips of citrus zest, minced

3 tablespoons sugar

3 tablespoons unsalted butter

Directions:

1. Put the juice in a small deep cooking pan. Over moderate to high heat, reduce the liquid by half.

2. Take away the pan from the heat and mix in the sugar and butter. Mix in the egg until well blended.

3. Return the pan to the burner and cook on medium-low heat for three to five minutes or until bubbles barely start to form.

4. Take away the pan from the heat and mix in the citrus zest. Put the pan in a container of ice and stir the mixture until it is cold.

5. In another container, whip the cream until firm. Fold the citrus mixture meticulously into the cream.

Yield: Servings 4

COCONUT CUSTARD

Ingredients:

1 (16-ounce) can coconut cream

3 tablespoons butter

6 big eggs, lightly beaten

1 cup fine granulated sugar

Fresh tropical fruit (not necessary)

Directions:

1. In a large, heavy-bottomed deep cooking pan, mix together the coconut cream and the sugar.

2. Over moderate heat, cook and stir the mixture until the sugar is thoroughly blended.

3. Lower the heat to low and mix in the eggs. Cook while stirring once in a while, until the mixture is thick and coats the back of a spoon, approximately ten to twelve minutes.

4. Take away the pan from the heat and put in the butter. Stir until the butter is completely melted and blended.

5. Pour the custard into six 4-ounce custard cups. Put the cups in a baking pan. Pour boiling water into the baking pan until it comes midway up the sides of the custard cups.

6. Cautiously move the baking pan to a preheated 325-degree oven. Bake the custards for thirty to forty minutes until set. (The tip of a knife should come out clean when inserted into the middle of the custard.)

7. Serve warm or at room temperature. Decorate using chopped

tropical fruit, if you wish.

Yield: Servings 6

COCONUT-PINEAPPLE SOUFFLÉ FOR 2

Ingredients:

½ cup (½-inch) cubes ladyfingers or sponge cake

1 egg yolk

2 egg whites

2 tablespoons dark rum

2 tablespoons finely chopped fresh pineapple

2 tablespoons sugar

2½ tablespoons grated sweetened coconut Lemon juice

Softened butter for the molds

Sugar for the molds

Directions:

16

1. Preheat your oven to 400 degrees.

2. Butter 2-¾ or 1-cup soufflée molds and then drizzle them with sugar. Place in your fridge the molds until ready to use.

3. Put the ladyfinger cubes in a small container. Pour the rum over the cubes and allow to soak for five minutes.

4. Squeeze the juice from the pineapple, saving both the pulp and 1 tablespoon of the juice.

5. In a small container, beat the egg yolk with the pineapple juice until very thick. Fold in the cake cubes, pineapple pulp, and coconut.

6. In another small container, beat the egg whites with a few drops of lemon juice until foamy. Slowly put in the 2 tablespoons of sugar, while continuing to beat until the whites are stiff and shiny.

7. Lightly fold the pineapple mixture into the egg whites.

8. Ladle the batter into the prepared molds and bake for eight to ten minutes or until puffy and mildly browned.

Yield: 2

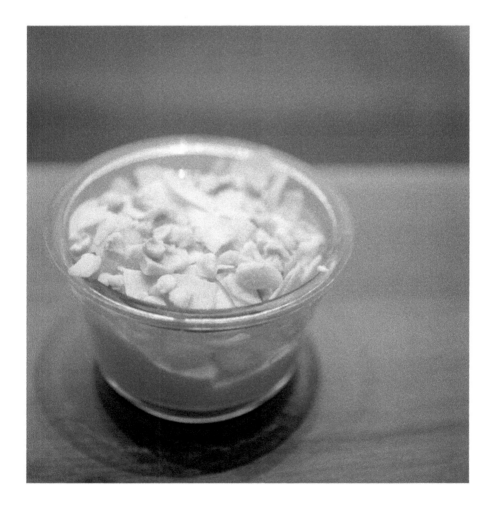

CRISPY CREPES WITH FRESH FRUIT

Ingredients:

¼ cup shredded, unsweetened coconut 1 cup heavy cream

1 package frozen puff pastry sheets, thawed in accordance with package instructions

1 tablespoon unflavored rum or coconut-flavored rum

2 cups raspberries, blueberries, or other fresh fruit, the best 12 berries reserved for decoration

2 tablespoons confectioner's sugar, divided

Directions:

1. Preheat your oven to 400 degrees.

2. Put the puff pastry sheet on a work surface and slice into 12 equalsized pieces. Put the pastry pieces on a baking sheet.

3. Bake the pastry roughly ten minutes. Take out of the oven and use a sifter to shake a small amount of the confectioner?s sugar over the puff pastry. Return to the oven and carry on baking for roughly five minutes or until golden. Put the puff pastry on a wire rack and let cool completely.

4. Put the berries in a food processor and for a short period of time process to make a rough purée.

5. Whip the cream with the rest of the confectioner's sugar until thick, but not firm. Mix in the coconut and the rum.

6. To serve, place 1 piece of puff pastry in the center of each serving plate, spoon some cream over the pastry, and then top with some purée. Put another pastry on top, decorate with some of the rest of the berries, any remaining juice from the purée,

and a drizzle of confectioner's sugar.

FRESH ORANGES IN ROSE WATER

Ingredients:

1½ cups sugar

3 cups water

4–6 teaspoons rose water

8 oranges

Directions:

1. Peel and segment the oranges. Put them in a container, cover, and set aside in your fridge.

2. In a deep cooking pan, bring the water and the sugar to its boiling point over moderatehigh heat. Boil gently for fifteen to 20 or until the mixture becomes syrupy. Turn off the heat and mix in the rose water. Allow to cool to room temperature and then place in your fridge

3. To serve, place orange segments in individual dessert cups. Pour rose water syrup over the top.

Yield: Servings 6–8

LEMONGRASS CUSTARD

Ingredients:

½ cup suga

2 cups whole milk

2 stalks fresh lemongrass, finely chopped (soft inner portion only)

6 egg yolks

Directions:

1. Preheat your oven to 275 degrees.

2. In a moderate-sized-sized deep cooking pan, on moderate to high heat, bring the milk and the lemongrass to its boiling point. Lower the heat and simmer for five minutes. Cover the milk mixture, remove the heat, and allow it to sit for about ten minutes on the burner.

3. In a mixing container, beat the egg yolks with the sugar until thick.

4. Strain the milk mixture through a fine-mesh sieve, then slowly pour it into the egg yolks, whisking continuously.

5. Split the mixture between 6 small custard cups and put the cups in a high-sided baking or roasting pan. Put in warm water to the pan so that it reaches to roughly an inch below the top of the custard cups. Cover the pan firmly using foil.

6. Put the pan in your oven and bake for roughly twenty minutes or until the custards are set on the sides but still slightly wobbly in the middle.

Yield: Servings 6

MANGO FOOL

Ingredients:

¼ cup sugar

1 cup heavy cream

1 tablespoon confectioners' sugar

2 ripe mangoes, peeled and flesh cut from the pits 2 tablespoons lime juice

Crystallized ginger (not necessary)

Mint leaves (not necessary)

Directions:

1. Put the mangoes in a food processor with the lime juice and sugar. Puréee until the desired smoothness is achieved.

2. In a big container beat the heavy cream with the confectioners' sugar until firm.

3. Thoroughly fold the mango purée into the heavy cream.

4. Serve in goblets decorated with crystallized ginger or sprigs of mint, if you wish.

Yield: Servings 4–6

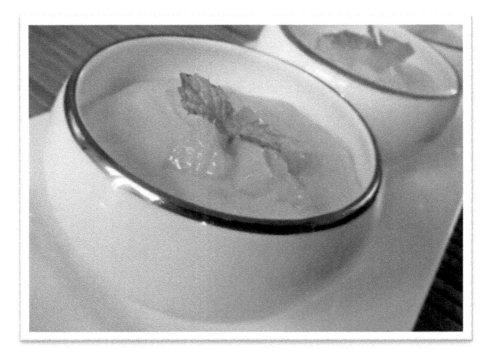

MANGO SAUCE OVER ICE CREAM

Ingredients:

1 banana, peeled and chopped

1 tablespoon brandy (not necessary)

2 mangoes, peeled, pitted, and diced

1 cup (or to taste) sugar

Juice of 2 big limes (or to taste)

Vanilla ice cream

Directions:

1. In a moderate-sized-sized deep cooking pan using low heat, simmer the mangoes, banana, sugar, and lime juice for thirty minutes, stirring regularly.

2. Put in the brandy and simmer 5 more minutes.

3. Turn off the heat and let cool slightly or to room temperature.

4. To serve, scoop ice cream into individual serving bowls. Ladle sauce over top.

Yield: 2 cups

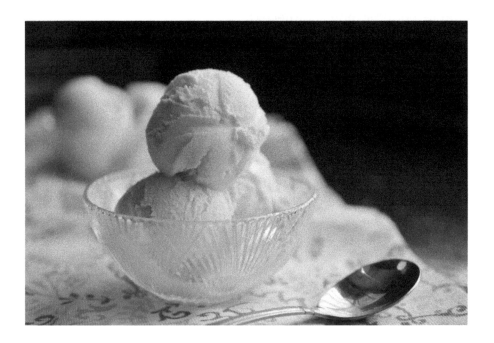

PINEAPPLE RICE

Ingredients:

¼ cup sugar

½ cup short-grained rice

1 ripe pineapple

2 teaspoons chopped crystallized ginger, divided

3 tablespoons roasted cashew nuts, chopped Pinch of salt

Zest and juice of 1 lemon

Directions:

1. Chop the pineapple in half along the length, leaving the leaves undamaged on 1 side. Scoop out the pineapple flesh of both halves, leaving a ½-inch edge on the half with the leaves. Dice the pineapple fruit from 1 half and purée the fruit from the other

half in a food processor together with the sugar and salt; set aside.

2. Strain the fruit purée through a fine-mesh sieve into a measuring cup. Put in enough water to make 1¾ cups. Move to a small deep cooking pan and bring to its boiling point on moderate to high heat.

3. Wash and drain the rice. Mix the rice into the pineapple purée. Mix in the lemon zest, lemon juice, and 1 teaspoon of the ginger. Bring to its boiling point; reduce heat, cover, and simmer until the liquid has been absorbed, approximately twenty minutes.

4. Combine the reserved pineapple cubes into the rice.

5. To serve, spoon the rice into the hollowed out pineapple that has the leaves. Decorate using the rest of the ginger and the roasted cashews.

Yield: Servings 4–6

PINEAPPLE-MANGO SHERBET

Ingredients:

½ cup plain yogurt

1 big orange, peeled and segmented

1 cup pineapple pieces

1 tablespoon lime zest

1 teaspoon orange-flavored liqueur (not necessary)

2 mangoes, peeled, pitted, and slice into 1-inch cubes

1 cup sugar

Directions:

1. Put the orange segments, mango cubes, and pineapple pieces on a baking sheet lined with waxed paper; store in your freezer for 30 to forty-five minutes or until just frozen.

2. Move the fruit to a food processor. Put in the lime zest and sugar, and pulse until well blended.

3. While the machine runs, add the yogurt and liqueur. Process for another three minutes or until the mixture is fluffy.

4. Pour the mixture into an 8" × 8" pan, cover using foil, and freeze overnight.

5. To serve, let the sherbet temper at room temperature for ten to fifteen minutes, then scoop into glass dishes.

Yield: Servings 4–6

PUMPKIN CUSTARD

Ingredients:

1 small cooking pumpkin

5 eggs

1 cup brown sugar

Directions:

1. With a small sharp knife, cautiously chop the top off of the pumpkin.

2. Using a spoon, remove and discard the seeds and most of the tender flesh; set the pumpkin aside.

3. In a moderate-sized-sized mixing container, whisk the eggs together. Mix in the brown sugar, salt, and coconut cream until well blended.

4. Pour the mixture into the pumpkin.

5. Put the pumpkin in a steamer and allow to steam for roughly twenty minutes or until the custard is set.

Yield: Servings 4

PUMPKIN SIMMERED IN COCONUT MILK

Ingredients:

½ cup coconut milk

½ teaspoon salt

1 cup water

2 cups fresh pumpkin meat cut into big julienned pieces (acorn squash is a good substitute)

1 cup brown sugar

Directions:

1. Place the water and the coconut milk in a moderate-sized pan using low heat. Put in the salt and half of the sugar; stir until well blended. Adjust the sweetness to your preference by put in more water or sugar if required.

2. Put in the julienned pumpkin to the pan and bring to its boiling point on moderate heat. Reduce to a simmer and cook until soft, approximately 5 to ten minutes depending on both the texture of the pumpkin and your own preference.

3. The pumpkin may be served hot, warm, or cold.

Yield: Servings 4

STEAMED COCONUT CAKES

Ingredients:

¼ cup all-purpose flour

½ cup coconut milk

½ cup grated sweet coconut

½ cup rice flour

4 tablespoons finely granulated sugar

5 eggs

Pinch of salt

Directions:

1. In a big mixing container, beat the eggs and the sugar together until thick and pale in color.

2. Put in the rice flours and salt.

3. Beating continuously, slowly pour in the coconut milk. Beat the batter for 3 more minutes.

4. Bring some water to boil in a steamer big enough to hold 10 small ramekins. When the water starts to boil, put the ramekins in the steamer to heat for a couple of minutes.

5. Split the shredded coconut uniformly between all of the ramekins and use a spoon to compact it on the bottom of the cups.

6. Pour the batter uniformly between the cups. Steam for about ten minutes.

7. Take away the cakes from the cups the moment they are sufficiently cool to handle.

8. Serve warm or at room temperature.

Yield: 10 cakes

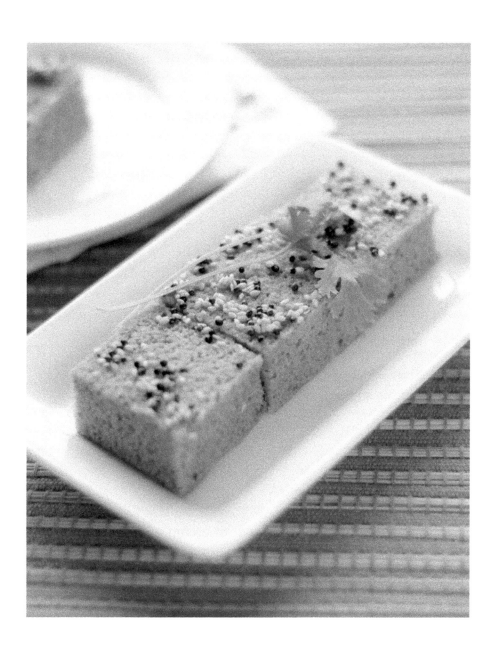

STICKY RICE WITH COCONUT CREAM SAUCE

Ingredients:

1 cup coconut cream

1 teaspoon salt

3 cups cooked Sweet Sticky Rice

4 ripe mangoes, thinly cut (or other tropical fruits)

4 tablespoons sugar

Directions:

1. For the sauce, put the coconut cream, sugar, and salt in a small deep cooking pan. Stir to blend and bring to its boiling point on moderate to high heat. Decrease the heat and simmer for five minutes.

2. To serve, position mango slices on each plate. Put a mound of rice next to the fruit. Top the rice with some of the sauce.

Yield: Servings 6

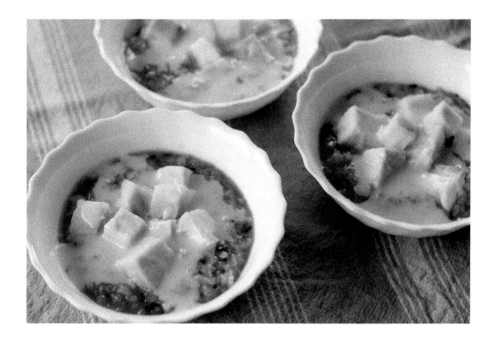

SWEET STICKY RICE

Ingredients:

½ cup granulated sugar

½ teaspoon salt

1 cups canned coconut milk

1½ cups white glutinous rice

Directions:

1. Put the rice in a container and put in enough water to completely cover the rice. Soak for minimum 4 hours or overnight. Drain.

2. Coat a steamer basket with wet cheesecloth. Spread the rice

uniformly over the cheesecloth. Put the container over quickly boiling water. Cover and steam until soft, approximately twenty-five minutes; set aside.

3. In a moderate-sized-sized deep cooking pan, mix the coconut milk, sugar, and salt and heat on moderate to high. Stir until the sugar is thoroughly blended. Pour over the rice, stir until blended, and allow to rest for half an hour

4. To serve, place in small bowls or on plates. Decorate using mangoes, papayas, or other tropical fruit.

Yield: Servings 6

TARO BALLS POACHED IN COCONUT MILK

Ingredients:

1 cup brown sugar

1 cup cooked taro, mashed

1 cup corn flour

2 cups glutinous rice flour

4 cups coconut milk

Fresh tropical fruit (not necessary)

teaspoon salt

Directions:

1. In a big mixing container, mix the rice and the flours.

2. Put in the mashed taro and knead to make a tender dough.

3. Roll into little bite-sized balls and save for later.

4. In a moderate-sized to big deep cooking pan, heat the coconut milk using low heat.

5. Put in the brown sugar and the salt, stirring until blended.

6. Bring the mixture to a low boil and put in the taro balls.

7. Poach the balls for five to ten minutes or until done to your preference.

8. Serve hot in small glass bowls, decorated with tropical fruit.

Yield: Servings 6–12

TOFU WITH SWEET GINGER

Ingredients:

1 (2- to 3-inch) piece of ginger, peeled and smashed using the back of a knife

1 12-ounce package tender tofu

3 cups water

1 cup brown sugar

Directions:

1. Put the water, ginger, and brown sugar in a small deep cooking pan. Bring to its boiling point using high heat. Lower the heat to a simmer and allow the sauce to cook for minimum ten minutes. (The longer you allow the mixture to cook, the spicier it will get.)

2. To serve, spoon some of the tofu into dessert bowls and pour some sauce over the top. (This sauce is equally good over plain yogurt.)

Yield: 3 cups of sauce

TROPICAL COCONUT RICE

Ingredients:

¼ cup toasted coconut

1 cup coconut cream

2 cups short-grained rice

2 cups water

Directions:

1. Place the rice, water, and coconut cream in a moderate-sized deep cooking pan and mix thoroughly. Bring to its boiling point on moderate to high heat. Decrease the heat and cover with a tight-fitting lid. Cook for fifteen to twenty minutes or until all of the liquid has been absorbed.

2. Allow the rice rest off the heat for five minutes.

3. Fluff the rice and mix in the toasted coconut and fruit.

Yield: Servings 6–8

TROPICAL FRUIT WITH GINGER CREÈME ANGLAISE

Ingredients:

(1-inch) pieces peeled gingerroot, slightly mashed 1 cup half-and-half

2 tablespoons sugar A variety of tropical fruits, cut

3 egg yolks

Directions:

1. In a small heavy deep cooking pan on moderate to low heat, bring the ginger and the half-and-half to a slight simmer. Do not boil.

2. Meanwhile, whisk together the eggs yolks and the sugar.

3. Slowly pour the hot half-and-half into the egg mixture, stirring continuously so that the eggs do not cook.

4. Pour the custard back into the deep cooking pan and cook on moderate to low heat, stirring continuously using a wooden spoon for five minutes or until slightly thickened.

5. Pour the crèmes anglaise through a mesh strainer into a clean container and let cool completely.

6. Pour over slices of your favorite tropical fruits.

Yield: 1½ cups

WATERMELON ICE

Ingredients:

½ cup sugar

1 (3-pound) piece of watermelon, rind cut away, seeded, and cut into little chunks (reserve a small amount for decoration if you wish)

1 cup water

1 tablespoon lime juice

Mint sprigs (not necessary)

Directions:

1. Put the water and sugar in a small deep cooking pan and bring to its boiling point. Turn off the heat and let cool to room temperature, stirring regularly. Set the pan in a container of ice and continue to stir the syrup until cold.

2. Put the watermelon, syrup, and lime juice in a blender and purée until the desired smoothness is achieved.

3. Pour the purée through a sieve into a 9-inch baking pan. Cover the pan using foil.

4. Put into your freezer the purée for eight hours or until frozen.

5. To serve, scrape the frozen purée with the tines of a fork. Ladle the scrapings into pretty glass goblets and decorate with a small piece of watermelon or mint sprigs.

Yield: Servings 6–8

FRESH COCONUT JUICE

Ingredients:

1 young coconut

Ice

Sprig of mint for decoration

Directions:

1. Using a meat cleaver, make a V-shaped slice on the top of the coconut.

2. Pour the juice over a glass of ice.

3. Decorate using a mint sprig.

Yield: Servings 1–2 depending on the size of the coconut.

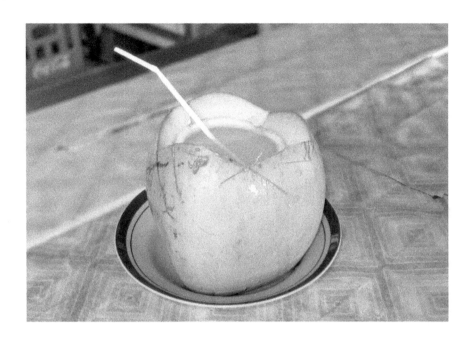

GINGER TEA

Ingredients:

½-¾ cup sugar

1 big branch (roughly

8 cups water

pound) of ginger, cut into long pieces

Directions:

1. Bring the water to its boiling point in a big pan. Put in the ginger, reduce heat, and simmer for ten to twenty minutes, depending on how strong you prefer your tea.

2. Take away the ginger and put in the sugar to taste, stirring until

it is thoroughly blended.

3. Serve hot or over ice.

Yield: 8 cups

ICED SWEET TEA

Ingredients:

1 cup hot water

1 tablespoon sugar

1 tablespoon sweetened condensed milk

1 teaspoon milk

1–2 tablespoons Thai tea leaves

Ice

Directions:

1. Place the sugar and sweetened condensed milk into a big glass.

2. Put the tea leaves into a tea ball and place it in the glass.

3. Put in the hot water. Allow to steep until done to your preferred strength.

4. Stir to dissolve the sugar and sweetened condensed milk.

5. Put in ice and top with milk.

Yield: slightly more than 1 cup.

LEMONGRASS TEA

Ingredients:

¼ – cup sugar

1 cup lemongrass stalks, chopped

8 cups water

Directions:

1. Bring the water to its boiling point in a big pan. Put in the lemongrass, turn off the heat, and allow to steep for ten to twenty minutes, depending on how strong you prefer your tea.

2. Take away the lemongrass and put in the sugar to taste, stirring until it is thoroughly blended.

3. Serve hot or over ice.

Yield: 8 cups

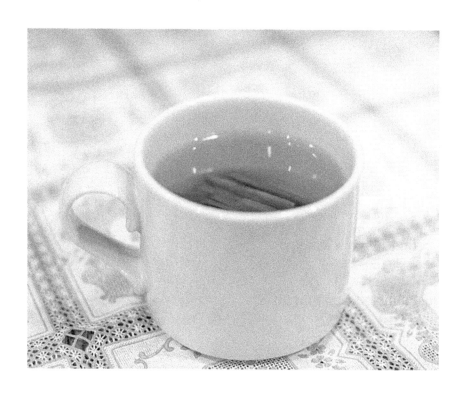

MANGO BELLINI

Ingredients:

½ teaspoon lemon juice

1 teaspoon mango schnapps

2 tablespoons puréed mango

Chilled champagne

Directions:

1. Put the mango purée, mango schnapps, and lemon juice in a champagne flute.

2. Fill the flute with champagne and stir.

Yield: 1 glass

ROYAL THAI KIR

Ingredients:

1–2 teaspoons creème de mango or mango schnapps Chilled dry champagne

Directions:

1. Pour the creème into a champagne flute and fill with champagne.

Yield: 1 glass

SUPER-SIMPLE THAI ICED TEA

Ingredients:

2 tablespoons sugar

1 cup hot water

Ice

1–2 tablespoons Thai tea leaves

Directions:

1. Place the sugar into a big glass.

2. Put the tea leaves in a tea ball and place it in the glass.

3. Put in the hot water. Allow to steep until done to your preferred strength.

4. Stir to dissolve the sugar and put in ice.

Yield: Approximately 1 cup

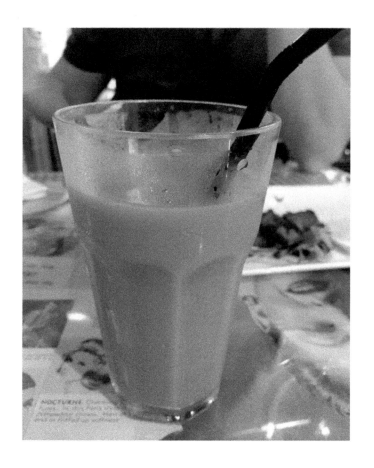

THAI "MARTINIS"

Ingredients:

1 bottle coconut rum

1 bottle dark rum

1 bottle light rum

1 whole ripe pineapple

3 stalks lemongrass, trimmed, cut into 3-inch lengths and tied in a bundle

Directions:

1. Take away the pineapple greens and then quarter the rest of the fruit. Put the pineapple quarters and the lemongrass bundle in a container big enough to hold all of the liquor.

2. Pour the rums over the fruit and stir until blended. Cover the container and let infuse for minimum one week at room temperature.

3. Take away the lemongrass bundle and discard.

4. Take away the pineapple quarters and slice into slices for decoration.

5. To serve, pour some of the rum into a martini shaker filled with ice; shake thoroughly. Pour into martini glasses and decorate with a pineapple slice.

Yield: 3 quarts

THAI ICED TEA

Ingredients:

1 cup sugar

1 cup Thai tea leaves

1–1½ cups half-and-half

6 cups water

Ice

Directions:

1. Bring the water to boil in a moderate-sized pot. Turn off the heat and put in the tea leaves, pushing them into the water until they are completely submerged. Steep roughly five minutes or until the liquid is a bright orange.

2. Strain through a fine-mesh sieve or coffee strainer.

3. Mix in the sugar until thoroughly blended.

4. Allow the tea to reach room temperature and then place in your

 fridge

5. To serve, pour the tea over ice cubes, leaving room at the top of the glass to pour in three to 4 tablespoons of half-and-half; stir for a short period of time to blend.

Yield: Approximately 8 cups

THAI LIMEADE

Ingredients:

1–½ cup sugar

1 cup lime juice, lime rinds reserved

8 cups water

Salt to taste (not necessary)

Directions:

1. Mix the lime juice and the sugar; set aside.

2. Bring the water to boil in a big pot. Put in the lime rinds and turn off the heat. Allow to steep for ten to fifteen minutes. Take away the lime rinds.

3. Put in the lime juice mixture to the hot water, stirring to completely dissolve the sugar. Put in salt if you wish.

4. Serve over ice.

Yield: 9 cups

THAI-INSPIRED SINGAPORE SLING

Ingredients:

¼– cup pineapple juice Mint sprig (not necessary)

1 tablespoon cherry brandy

1 tablespoon lime juice

1 tablespoon orange liqueur

1 teaspoon brown sugar

2 tablespoons whiskey

Dash of bitters

Directions:

1. Put all of the ingredients into a cocktail shaker and shake thoroughly to blend.

2. Serve over crushed ice and decorate with a sprig of mint if you wish.

Yield: 1 cocktail

TROPICAL FRUIT COCKTAIL

Ingredients:

1 small mango, papaya, banana, or other tropical fruit, peeled and roughly chopped (reserve a small amount for decoration if you wish)

1 tablespoon brown sugar

1 teaspoon grated ginger

1⁄ cups orange or grapefruit juice

1⁄ cups pineapple juice

1–½ cup (or to taste) rum

4 tablespoons lime or lemon juice

Directions:

1. Put the chopped fruit, lime juice, ginger, and sugar in a blender and process until the desired smoothness is achieved.

2. Put in the rest of the ingredients to the blender and pulse until well blended.

3. To serve, pour over crushed ice and garnish with fruit slices of your choice.

Yield: 3–4 cups

ALMOND "TEA"

Ingredients:

¼–½ cup sugar

½ teaspoon ground cardamom

2 cups milk

2 ounces pumpkin seeds

3 cups water

3 ounces blanched almonds

Directions:

1. Process the almonds, pumpkin seeds, cardamom, and half of the water in a blender or food processor until the solids are thoroughly ground.

2. Strain the almond water through cheesecloth (or a clean Handi Wipe) into a container. Using the back of a spoon, press the solids to remove as much moisture as you can.

3. Return the almond mixture to the blender and put in the remaining water. Process until meticulously blended.

4. Strain this liquid into the container.

5. Mix the milk into the almond water. Put in sugar to taste.

6. Serve over crushed ice.

Yield: Servings 4–6

BANANA BROWN RICE PUDDING

Ingredients:

¼ cup water

½ teaspoon cinnamon

½ teaspoon nutmeg

1 (fifteen-ounce) can fruit cocktail, drained

1 cup skim milk

1 medium banana, cut

1 teaspoon vanilla extract

1½ cups cooked brown rice

2 tablespoons honey

Directions:

1. In a moderate-sized-sized deep cooking pan, mix the banana, fruit cocktail, water, honey, vanilla, cinnamon, and nutmeg. Bring to its boiling point on moderate to high heat. Lower the heat and simmer for about ten minutes or until the bananas are soft.

2. Mix in the milk and the rice. Return the mixture to its boiling point, decrease the heat again, and simmer for ten more minutes. Serve warm.

Yield: Servings 4–6

CARDAMOM COOKIES

Ingredients:

½ cup fine sugar

1 cup fine semolina

1½ teaspoons ground cardamom

3 tablespoons all-purpose flour

4 ounces ghee

Directions:

1. Preheat your oven to 300 degrees.

2. In a big mixing container, cream together the ghee and the sugar until light and fluffy.

3. Sift together the semolina, all-purpose flour, and cardamom.

4. Mix the dry ingredients into the ghee mixture; mix thoroughly.

5. Allow the dough stand in a cool place for half an hour

6. Form balls using roughly 1 tablespoon of dough for each. Put on an ungreased cookie sheet and flatten each ball slightly.

7. Bake for roughly thirty minutes or until pale brown.

8. Cool on a wire rack. Store in an airtight container.

Yield: 2 dozen cookies

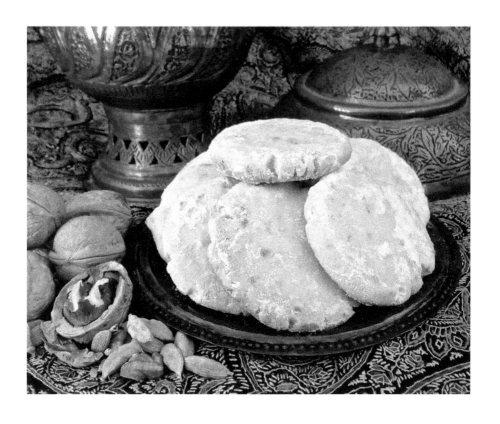

82

CHAPATI

Ingredients:

1 cup lukewarm water

1 tablespoon ghee or oil

1½ teaspoons salt

3 cups whole-wheat flour

Directions:

1. In a big mixing container, mix together 2½ cups of flour and the salt. Put in the ghee and, using your fingers, rub it into the flour and salt mixture.

2. Put in the lukewarm water and mix to make a dough. Knead the dough until it is smooth and elastic, approximately ten minutes. (Do not skimp on the kneading; it is what makes the bread soft.)

3. Form the dough into a ball and put it in a small, oiled container. Cover firmly using plastic wrap and allow it to rest at room temperature for minimum 1 hour.

4. Split the dough into golf ball–sized pieces. Using a flour-covered rolling pin, roll each ball out on a flour-covered surface to roughly 6 to 8 inches in diameter and -inch thick.

5. Heat a big frying pan or griddle on moderate heat. Put a piece of dough on the hot surface. Using a towel or the edge of a spoon, cautiously press down around the edges of the bread. (This will allow air pockets to make in the bread.) Cook for a minute.

Cautiously turn the chapati over and carry on cooking for 1 more minute. Chapatis must be mildly browned and flexible, not crunchy. Take away the bread to a basket and cover using a towel. Repeat until all of the rounds are cooked.

Yield: Servings 6–8

CHILIED COCONUT DIPPING SAUCE

Ingredients:

¼ cup fresh coconut juice

1 serrano chili, seeded and minced

1 tablespoon lime juice

1 teaspoon rice wine vinegar

1 teaspoon sugar

2 cloves garlic, minced

2 tablespoons fish sauce

Directions:

1. Bring the coconut juice, rice wine vinegar, and sugar to its boiling point in a small deep cooking pan. Turn off the heat and allow the mixture to cool completely.

2. Mix in the rest of the ingredients.

Yield: Approximately 1 cup

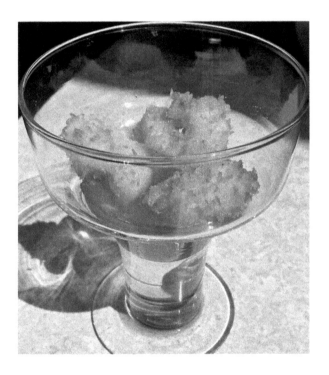

CUCUMBER RAITA

Ingredients:

1 teaspoon salt

1½ cups plain yogurt

1–2 green onions, trimmed and thinly cut

2 seedless cucumbers, peeled and slice into a small dice

2 tablespoons fresh mint

Lemon juice to taste

Directions:

1. Put the diced cucumbers in a colander. Drizzle with salt and allow it to sit in the sink for fifteen minutes to drain. Wash the

cucumber under cold water and drain once more.

2. Mix the cucumber, yogurt, green onions, mint, and lemon juice to taste.

3. Cover and place in your fridge for minimum 30 minutes. Check seasoning, putting in additional salt and/or lemon juice if required.

Yield: Approximately 4 cups

FRUIT IN SHERRIED SYRUP

Ingredients:

1 orange, peeled and segmented

1½ cups kiwi slices

2 cups fresh pineapple chunks

2 tablespoons dry sherry

2 tablespoons sugar

2 teaspoons lemon juice

4 tablespoons water

Directions:

1. In a small deep cooking pan using high heat, boil the sugar and the water until syrupy. Turn off the heat and let cool completely. Mix in the lemon juice and sherry; set aside.

2. In a serving container, mix the orange segments, the pineapple chunks, and the kiwi. Pour the syrup over the fruit and toss to blend. Place in your fridge for minimum 1 hour before you serve.

Yield: Servings 4–6

GARAM MASALA

Ingredients:

1 tablespoon whole black peppercorns

1 teaspoon whole cloves

2 small cinnamon sticks, broken into pieces

2 tablespoons cumin seeds

2 teaspoons cardamom seeds

4 tablespoons coriander seeds

Directions:

1. In a small heavy sauté pan, individually dry roast each spice on moderate to high heat until they start to release their aroma.
2. Allow the spices to cool completely and then put them in a spice grinder and process to make a quite fine powder.

3. Store in an airtight container.

Yield: Approximately 1 cup

HAPPY PANCAKES

Ingredients:

¼ cup mixed, chopped herbs (mint, cilantro, basil, etc.)

¼ teaspoon salt

½ cup bean sprouts

½ cup finely cut straw mushrooms, washed and patted dry 1 cup rice flour

1 tablespoon vegetable oil

1 teaspoon sugar

1½ cups water

2 eggs, lightly beaten

3 ounces cooked salad shrimp, washed and patted dry Chili dipping sauce

Directions:

1. In a moderate-sized-sized container, whisk together the rice

flour, water, eggs, salt, and sugar. Set aside and let the batter rest for about ten minutes.

2. Strain the batter through a mesh sieve to remove any lumps.

3. Put in the vegetable oil to a big sauté or omelet pan. Heat on high until super hot, but not smoking.

4. Pour the batter into the hot pan, swirling it so that it coats the bottom of the pan uniformly. Drizzle the mushrooms over the batter. Cover and allow to cook for a minute.

5. Drizzle the shrimp and bean sprouts uniformly over the pancake. Carry on cooking until the bottom is crunchy and browned.

6. To serve, chop the pancake into four equivalent portions. Drizzle with the chopped herbs. Pass a favorite dipping sauce separately.

Yield: Servings 4

LIME

Ingredients:

½ teaspoon sesame oil

½–1 teaspoon cinnamon Pinch of salt

3 tablespoons honey

6 cups of tropical fruits, such as mango, papaya, bananas, melons, star fruit, kiwi, etc., (anything really) cut into bite-sized pieces

Zest and juice of 6 limes

Directions:

1. Mix the lime zest and all but about of the lime juice in a small container. Slowly sprinkle in the honey, whisking to make a smooth mixture. Whisk in the sesame oil, cinnamon, and salt. Adjust flavor to your preference with more lime juice if required.

2. Put the fruit in a big serving container. Pour the cinnamon-lime dressing over the fruit, toss to blend, and allow to rest in your fridge for fifteen minutes before you serve.

Yield: Servings 6–12

VIETNAMESE BANANAS

Ingredients:

1 tablespoon grated ginger Grated zest of 1 orange

3 tablespoons brown sugar

3 tablespoons butter

3 tablespoons shredded coconut (unsweetened)

3 teaspoons toasted sesame seeds

4 tablespoons lime juice

6 bananas, peeled and cut in half along the length

6 tablespoons orange liqueur

Directions:

1. Heat a small nonstick pan using high heat. Put in the coconut and cook, stirring continuously, until a golden-brown colour is achieved. Take away the coconut from the pan and save for later.

2. In a big sauté pan, melt the butter on moderate to high heat. Mix in the brown sugar, the ginger, and orange zest. Put the bananas in the pan, cut-side down, and cook for one to two minutes or until the sauce begins to become sticky. Turn the bananas over to coat in the sauce. Put the bananas on a heated serving platter and cover using aluminium foil.

3. Return the pan to the heat and meticulously mix in the lime juice and the orange liqueur. Using a long-handled match, ignite the sauce. Allow the flames to die down and then pour the sauce over the bananas.

4. Drizzle the bananas with the toasted coconut and the sesame seeds. Serve instantly.

Yield: Servings 6

VIETNAMESE OXTAIL SOUP

Ingredients:

¼ cup chopped cilantro

½ pound bean sprouts

1 (7-ounce) package rice sticks, soaked in hot water until tender and drained

1 green onion, trimmed and thinly cut

1 small cinnamon stick

1 tablespoon vegetable oil

1 tablespoon whole black peppercorns

1 whole star anise

2 garlic cloves, peeled and crushed

2 limes, cut into wedges

2 medium carrots, peeled and julienned

2 medium onions

3 tablespoons fish sauce

4 (½-inch) pieces ginger, peeled

4 serrano chilies, seeded and thinly cut

5 pounds meaty oxtails

Freshly ground black pepper to taste

Directions:

1. Cut 1 of the onions into ¼-inch slices. Heat the vegetable oil in a moderate-sized sauté pan on moderate to high heat. Put in the onion slices and sauté until they barely start to brown. Drain the oil from the browned onion and save for later.

2. Slice the rest of the onion into paper-thin slices. Cover using plastic wrap and save for later.

3. Wash the oxtails in cold water and put them in a stock pot. Cover the tails with cold water and bring to its boiling point. Lower the heat and skim any residue that has come to the surface. Let simmer for fifteen minutes.

4. Put in the browned onions, ginger, carrots, cinnamon, star anise, peppercorns, and garlic. Return the stock to a simmer and cook for 6 to 8 hours, putting in water if required.

5. When the broth is done, skim off any additional residue. Take away the oxtails from the pot and allow to cool until easy to handle. Take away the meat from the bones. Position the meat on a platter and decorate it with the cut green onions. Discard the bones.

6. Strain the broth and return to the stove. Put in the fish sauce and black pepper to taste. Keep warm.

7. On a second platter, position the bean sprouts, chopped cilantro, cut chilies, and lime wedges.

8. Bring a pot of water to its boiling point. Plunge the softened rice noodles in the water to heat. Drain.

9. To serve, place a portion of the noodles in each container. Set a

tureen of the broth on the table together with the platter of oxtail meat and the platter of accompaniments. Let your guests serve themselves.

Yield: Servings 6–8

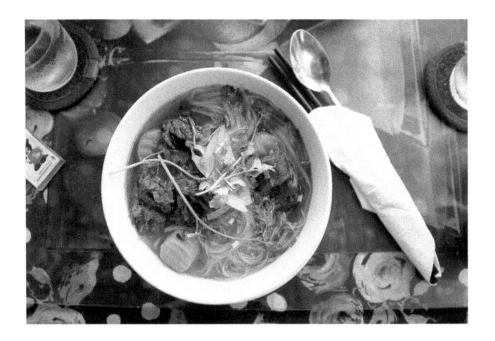

OMELET "EGG ROLLS"

Ingredients:

For the filling:

½ pound ground pork or chicken

½ teaspoon sugar

1 cup shredded Chinese cabbage

1 tablespoon fish sauce

1 tablespoon minced cilantro

1 teaspoon vegetable oil

2 green onions, trimmed and thinly cut

For the omelets:

1 tablespoon soy or fish sauce

1 teaspoon vegetable oil

6 tablespoons water

8 eggs

Bibb lettuce

Decorate of your choice

Soy sauce, fish sauce, and/or hot sauce

Directions:

1. To make the filling: In a moderate-sized-sized frying pan, warm the vegetable oil on moderate heat. Put in the ground meat and sauté until it is no longer pink. Put in the green onions and cabbage and cook until tender. Put in the sugar, fish sauce, and cilantro; cook for 1 more minute. Set the filling aside, keeping it warm.

2. To make the omelets: Mix the eggs, water, and soy sauce in a moderate-sized container. Put an omelet pan on moderate heat

for a minute. Put in roughly ¼ teaspoon of vegetable oil, swirling it to coat the pan uniformly. Pour roughly ¼ of the egg mixture into the pan, then allow it to rest for roughly half a minute. When the bottom is firm, flip the omelet and cook until done. Transfer to a plate and cover using foil to keep warm. Repeat to make 3 more omelets.

3. To fill the "Egg Rolls," place 1 omelet in the middle of a plate. Put ¼ of the filling slightly off-center and then roll up. Trim the ends and chop the rolls into bite-sized pieces.

4. To serve, use Bibb lettuce leaves to pick up the rolls. Immerse in additional soy sauce, fish sauce, hot sauce, or other favorite dipping sauce, and put in the decorate of your choice.

Yield: 16–20 pieces

VEGETABLES POACHED IN COCONUT MILK

Ingredients:

½ cup cut mushrooms

½ cup long beans or green beans, broken into two-inch pieces
½ cup peas

½ teaspoon cut kaffir lime leaves

1 cup coconut milk

1 cup shredded cabbage

1 shallot, finely chopped

1 tablespoon brown sugar

1 tablespoon green peppercorns, tied together in a small pouch

made from a Handi Wipe

1 tablespoon soy sauce

1 tablespoon Thai chilies, seeded and finely cut Rice, cooked in accordance with package directions

Directions:

1. In a deep cooking pan bring the coconut milk to a gentle simmer moderate heat. Mix in the shallots, soy sauce, brown sugar, green peppercorn pouch, and lime leaves. Simmer for 1 until aromatic.

2. Put in the green beans, mushrooms, and cabbage, and return simmer. Cook for five to ten minutes or until soft.

3. Put in the peas and cook 1 more minute. Take away the pouch before you serve over rice.

Yield: Servings 2–4

LEMON RICE

Ingredients:

¼ cup cashew nuts, soaked in cold water for five minutes

¼ teaspoon mustard seed

½ teaspoon turmeric

1 cup basmati rice, soaked in cold water for thirty minutes

1 cups water Pinch of salt

1 green chili pepper, seeded and minced

1 tablespoon vegetable oil

8 fresh curry leaves

Juice of ½ lemon

Directions:

1. In a moderate-sized-sized pan, bring the water to its boiling point. Put in the salt, rice, and turmeric; reduce heat, cover, and simmer for about ten minutes. (At the end of the ten minutes, the rice will have absorbed all of the liquid.) Turn off the heat and allow to cool.

2. In a wok, heat the oil and stir-fry the chili pepper. Put in the nuts, mustard seed, and curry leaves; carry on cooking for another half a minute. Mix in the lemon juice. Put in the cooled rice to the wok and toss until heated.

Yield: Servings 2–4

MANGO AND ICE CREAM

Ingredients:

1 banana, peeled and chopped

1 tablespoon brandy (not necessary)

2 mangoes, peeled, pitted, and diced

1 cup (or to taste) sugar

Vanilla ice cream

Directions:

1. In a moderate-sized-sized deep cooking pan using low heat, simmer the mangoes, banana, sugar, and lime juice for thirty minutes, stirring regularly.

2. Put in the brandy and simmer 5 more minutes.

3. Turn off the heat and let cool slightly or to room temperature.

4. To serve, scoop ice cream into individual serving bowls.

Yield: 2 cups

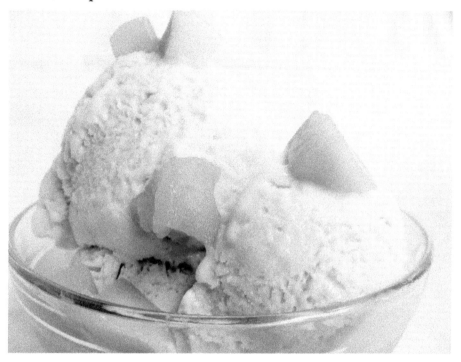

Lightning Source UK Ltd.
Milton Keynes UK
UKHW021833200421
382338UK00003B/291